How to Improve Posture

Achieve Perfect Posture with These 20 Easy Posture Correction Tips

by Cynthia D. Elliot

Table of Contents

Introduction

Most of us have noticed, at some point or another, that a person sitting with their head low and their hands on their cheeks is feeling sad, but that a person looking forward with his eyes sharp and his hands on his cheek is in deep thought. How did we come to such conclusions on first sight? It all has to do with how higher animals choose a prey from a herd. It's based on an involuntary notion called posture.

&

We express ourselves in a variety of different ways. These can be voluntary, in the form of language, gestures or art forms. However, we also involuntarily convey our inner thoughts to the people around us, through body language. People around you can read you like a book, especially if they know you well, or if they happen to be adept at the art of reading body language. It takes a long time and arduous practice to become a master in controlling one's own body language and to read the subtle body languages of the people around us.

Posture is the art of carrying oneself around. It may be while sitting, walking or even making a move; your posture tells people a lot about your thoughts, attitude and mood at that moment. Your posture is also the result of your physical fitness. In that way, it's actually a dual–component characteristic. Good physical health is needed to maintain good posture while good posture is necessary to maintain the proper functioning of various organ systems.

Maintaining good posture is an involuntary act. When your posture is not good, voluntary correction is needed in order to override your involuntary posture and replace it with a better posture. This needs persistent practice and continuous conscious correction of minute body language details. This book will take you through the fundamental facts about posture, the deleterious effects of bad posture, why it's necessary to maintain good posture and the effects of good posture on your body and mind. If you want to solve problems with your posture and generally improve the way you carry yourself, this is the book for you.

Tip #1: Identify the Problem

If you are unable unconsciously to maintain an erect posture while sitting or standing, it may point to some problems in your health. As the human body naturally tries to acquire the posture in which it is most comfortable, your posture may be due to an underlying problem which may cause pain or stress to the muscles and bones when you try to shift to an erect posture while sitting or standing. It is usually easy to find the faulty spot if you focus on the region where you feel a discomfort while maintaining a normal erect posture. If you are unable to find it, you can visit your physician to find and create a plan to solve the problem.

Tip #2: What is Good Posture?

Most of us are not aware of what good posture is, and thus are not sure if our posture is good or bad. To check this, stand sideways in front of a mirror. Stand with your chin lifted facing straight ahead, shoulders straight and widened, arms by the sides and with straight lower back with unbent knees. When you stand in this posture, your backbone will look like an S shaped curve with the backbone curving outward from neck to the beginning of hip region from where it curves inwards and extends to the lower back.

If your involuntary posture is different from this, try to maintain this alignment for a few minutes. If you are able to maintain it without any pain or discomfort, all you have to do is practice regularly to adapt to the right posture. If you have light discomfort, then it's time to give your muscles some exercise.

Tip #3: Strengthening Muscles

Good posture can be maintained only if the muscles are strong enough to support the bones properly. The major muscles involved in maintaining posture are the neck muscles, muscles of the back, and muscles around the hip. These muscles can be strengthened by giving them proper exercise. Let's begin with the neck muscles.

Tip #4: A Strong and Straight Neck

Stand or sit erect with your chin up. Turn your face to your left side and then to your right side. Repeat this 5 times on each side before coming back to the neutral position. Following this, bend your head backwards as far as you can go without exerting pressure, then bend forward so that your chin touches your chest. Repeat this 5 times and then come back to neutral. After this, rotate your head clockwise in such a way that your chin touches the shoulder edges and the chest like an arc. Repeat this 5 times and then do it in an anticlockwise direction and come back to neutral position. These simple exercises loosen up and strengthen the neck muscles so that the neck can be held upright for a long period of time.

Tip #5: Strengthen Your Shoulders

Stand with your feet apart. Raise both hands sideways to the level of your shoulder. Hold this to the count of 10 and then bring them back to neutral. Repeat this exercise 10 times. After doing this, raise your hands sideways, above your head, and let the palms touch each other like you are praying. Hold them in this position for 10 seconds and then bring them back to neutral. Repeat this exercise 10 times. These two exercises will strengthen the group of muscles around your shoulder joint and prevent you from stooping forward.

Tip #6: Strengthen Your Backbone

The back bone or spine is the key to maintaining good posture. It is the connection between the upper and lower parts of your body. People who have bad posture most commonly have problems in their spine. So let's go through some simple exercises which can make your spine strong and articular at the same time.

Stand with you feet apart. Place your hands on your hips as if you are holding your midsection. Bend forwards at the hip without bending your knees. After a few seconds, get back to a neutral position and then bend backwards as far as you can. It is important that you don't push too hard. Get back to neutral again. Repeat this to and fro exercise 10 times. Take 5 deep breaths after the exercise, then bend sideways to the left with your hands on your hips. Then get back to neutral and bend towards your right. Do this sideways bending 10 times and then get back to a neutral position. After a few deep breaths, rotate your hip slowly in a clockwise and anticlockwise direction in an imaginary hoola hoop. Rotate it 10 times in both directions. This exercise makes loosen up your hip muscles and make them capable of holding an erect, confident posture for a long period time and giving you a confident and springy gait.

Tip #7: Meditation

Apart from giving you inner peace, meditation helps a great deal in attaining good posture. Sit on a mat with your legs folded under you. Keep your back straight and close your eyes. Take deep and slow breaths and try to concentrate on the flow of air into and out of your body. Also focus on your body posture and feel the straightness of your back. Concentrate on pulling your breath deep into your body, all the way into your abdomen. Do this exercise for at least 10 minutes initially. You can increase the duration with regular practice.

Tip #8: Practicing Posture

Good posture portrays you outwardly to others as a confident person, while bad posture can give away your subconscious fears and insecurities. Let's do a little practice with your standing posture. We all have marked our heights on the walls when we were kids, right? Imagine that and stand close to a wall, in front of the mirror. Concentrate on your legs and the position of your backbone against the wall, keeping your head held high. Now stand in the middle of the room, in front of the mirror, and check out how long you can hold your posture as you did when you were with your back to the wall. Try to stand in this posture for 5 minutes initially and then increase the duration later. You can add a few alterations to the posture, like keeping your feet slightly apart and so on to look more casual.

Tip #9: Practice Walking

Good posture can make your gait attractive and cool. Keep your body relaxed and take the standing posture as above. Start walking leisurely with arms swinging at your sides slightly with each step. Avoid bending forward or taking faster steps, which makes you look hasty. Don't take your steps too high and don't take longer steps. The way you walk can indicate that you are on an urgent job, a casual walk, a relaxed stroll or a worried jaunt. It all depends on how you maintain your posture while walking.

Tip #10: Sitting Takes Practice

Are you aware of your posture while you sit in a chair? It can tell a lot about your inner personality or mood. Occupying just the edge of the chair with a stoop shoulders and arms on your legs means you lack confidence and are uncomfortable in that situation. You can take a neutral position by sitting in the chair with your back straight and feet touching the floor. The posture of confidence for women is to sit with your legs crossed at the knee with one of your arm resting on the armrest of the chair while your other hand rests on your lap. Make sure that your back is straight and lies against the back rest. Keep your shoulders square and straight and look ahead with confidence. This posture emits a positive attitude and is one of those first, impressive postures associated with any business deal, negotiation, or job interview. Once in a while, sit on the floor, taking up the meditation position, to practice the proper sitting posture.

Tip #11: Maintain or Change?

You may doubt how long you will be able to hold up your position either while sitting or standing. Don't worry. You don't need to maintain an erect posture like a statue for a long period of time. Change your postures regularly. If you have been sitting for half an hour, take a walk for a few minutes. You need not go outdoors to take this break. If you have been working on your laptop for quite a while, take a walk to pick up something on your table or go grab a glass of water from the break room kitchen.

Regardless of how good your posture is, if you have been sitting in the same position for a long time, it is going to damage your muscles. So change is good. Try to do some stretching exercises in the same spot if you are unable to leave your work place. Raise your right hand above your head and try to touch your left shoulder with your fingertips. Do this a few times and then do it with your left hand. This exercise will relax the shoulder muscles. Similarly, bend sideways out of the chair as if picking up an imaginary object from the floor. Use your right hand for your right side and your left hand for your left. Perform these exercises a couple of times to relax your hip muscles. You can do all the neck and shoulder strengthening muscles while sitting in your workplace if you feel that you have been glued in the same place for a long time.

Tip #12: Rising Posture

You need good posture not only to maintain your appearance when in the company of others, but also for good physical health. It's not uncommon to hear pain and sprain stories due to a faulty position in getting out of bed. It is always safe to turn to sideways before you get out of bed. Avoid getting up right away while you are on your back. People who do regular exercises and train their muscles for various stresses can cope with strain in any direction. But a normal person, who has very little habit of exercising, is more likely to have a muscle pull while getting out of bed in the wrong way. So always rise slowly from bed, sideways.

Tip #13: Want to Be a Sleeping Beauty?

Sleeping posture is very important for a peaceful and undisturbed sleep. Some people fall asleep wherever they are. It may be easy for them to fall asleep, but their bad posture will hurt after they wake up. You feel sleepy because your body and mind are tired. When you don't allow them to relax completely, you are not going to feel fresh after your sleep. Sleeping on a sofa with your legs dangling or sleeping while sitting in a chair is not the right way to relax your body and mind. Never train your body to fall asleep in positions other than lying supine. Lie down on a flat bed or mat so that your limbs are in line with your body. Keep the bed soft so that your back doesn't hurt. If you only feel comfortable when your head is slightly lifted, place a thin and soft pillow under your head. However, don't elevate your head too much because you will feel sore in your neck muscles in the morning. It's not a problem to sleep on your side, but it's unhealthy to sleep face down or with your face covered with a blanket. If you are not aware of your sleeping posture, just recall if there is any pain or discomfort in your body when you wake up after a good night's sleep. If there is, then it's time to change your sleeping posture.

Tip #14: Train Your Back Muscles

Try these simple exercises and practice them routinely to avoid a hunched back and stooping shoulders. Place a mat on the floor. Lie down with your belly touching the mat. Place your palms on the sides of your head and try to lift your upper body off the ground. Bend your shoulder and neck backwards as if looking at the sky. Then get back to a prone position on the mat. Repeat this exercise 5 times initially and then increase the numbers by regular practice.

Lie down on your back on the mat with your arms by the side of your body. Now twist your hip and move the lower half of your body to the left side. Try not to move the upper half of the body. Come back to neutral position and then twist the lower half of your body towards the right side. Repeat this exercise 5 times initially and then increase the numbers up to 20 with regular practice. This exercise helps a lot in maintaining an erect back.

Tip #15: Reinforce

Are you unable to maintain an erect posture voluntarily? Don't worry. There are easy reinforcing techniques to adapt your brain to the erect posture. Stand erect with your backbone straight. Take a soft, non-elastic, non-stretchable wide tape or cloth. Wind it from your left shoulder to the right side of hip bone on your back side. Similarly, wind the tape from your right shoulder to the left side of your hip bone, so that it looks like and X shape on your back. Ask for some assistance so that you can wind it tightly across your erect back, so that you are unable to bend or hunch easily. This helps to maintain the erect posture for a long time, which is then saved in the brain as a habitual posture. Use this technique regularly until your body and mind accept this posture as an inherent one and get adapted to the muscles' contraction or relaxation in this posture.

Reinforce yourself in a chin up posture. When you have to sit or stand without performing any job, try to focus on objects or an imaginary point slightly above the line of your straight line of vision. This makes you to sit with your chin up. Though this makes you feel funny initially, regular practice of this technique will make you to take up this posture involuntarily.

Tip #16: A Good Diet

Physical health comes down to maintaining a proper, healthy, nutritious diet. Though maintaining good posture looks like an idle job for the body, a large number of muscles have to work to keep your body straight and stable without abnormal and ridiculous movements. The energy for these bulky muscle groups comes from the food you eat. So plan to keep your diet wholesome. Make it a balanced diet, with ample amounts of carbohydrates in the form of tubers like potato, cassava and fruits, rice etc.; protein in the form of red meat, pulses and grains; essential fats in the form of fish and other sea foods. Apart from the major nutrients, taking plenty of colorful fruits helps to detoxify the dangerous chemicals produced by the muscles during their metabolism. Therefore, a good, nutritious and wholesome diet is the key to maintaining good posture.

Tip #17: Fresh Air and Game Play

Have you heard of the term "muscle memory" before? Well, it's true. Muscles have inherent memory in them. With practice at skills like typing, you can do them with your eyes closed, simply by the muscle memory of your hands and fingers. In a similar way, with proper practice, your posture will be stored in the memory of the muscles involved. For this to happen, these muscle groups must be put to constant use. Engage yourself in outdoor games like football, soccer, or hockey where you need to move constantly. This will help you not only to maintain good posture, but also to maintain a decent shape to your body as the excess fat is shed off. If you are unable to go out for sports and games, do same spot jogging and walking in your home. In this way, your muscles get toned up and will be in an active state, with the ability to cope with stress and strain.

Tip #18: Things to Remember

Nothing can happen overnight. Everything needs some time, and this is especially true when breaking faulty posture habits. So don't lose heart if you are unable to maintain good posture for a long period of time. Begin with focusing on your posture on and off. It may be tiring to constantly be aware that your body has taken up the faulty posture, correcting it on every occasion. But be persistent in correcting your posture as often as possible, even if it's annoying at the beginning. Motivate yourself. Indulge yourself after keeping a successful posture for a specific amount of time.

Bear in mind that, like all physical exercise, posture correction causes mild soreness and discomfort which will be relieved spontaneously with time and practice. If you feel very uncomfortable or intolerable pain, it means that you have an underlying problem in your muscles, nerves or bones. It's time to visit your physician. Don't try any more correction techniques without your physician's advice.

Tip #19: Dos and Don'ts

Never overdo anything. Fix a regular time and duration for the posture correction techniques. Avoid strenuous exercises without proper medical explanation, as it may cause more harm than good. There is no shortcut to success. So don't get into traps like miracle medicines and other things which are said to give glowing confidence and good posture. Remember that good posture does not require a perfect curvy shape. Posture is how you carry yourself, which can convey a lot about your mood and attitude at that very instant. Good posture can therefore make a person look confident and positive, regardless of their physical shape or superficial beauty. Try to move around more often, and avoid being in the same position for a long time. Once in a while, use the stairs instead of the elevator.

Tip #20: All in the Mind

Posture is never a voluntary act. The underlying notion in correcting faulty posture lies in saving the details of good posture as an involuntary message to the brain. This needs constant practice and motivation. Inspiration should come from within. Relax your mind with yoga, meditation, music or any form of art. Reinforce the thought that your mind is in control of your body and that you can make your body obey your thoughts. Never lose hope from initial setbacks in your exercise regimes. Your mental strength can do wonders if you train it well. Any hard exercise can be made easy if you do it in a fun way. That's the reason you have to engage yourself in sports and games. The benefits from sports are extensive. Not only do they keep your muscles constantly active, they also help you to shed excess fat and tighten up the flabby skin which can give you an aged and plump appearance.

Conclusion

Posture is just a tiny speck in the vast ocean of body language. The above techniques need to be practiced regularly for any positive change. Every change needs a well planned, holistic approach and persistent effort to achieve what you have in mind. Put in unrelenting, hard work and unbeatable faith in yourself and you can easily overcome the hurdles in achieving good posture. There is no doubt that when your posture becomes perfect, your confidence levels get an automatic boost, and your attitude takes a positive turn. Your appearance is the first thing that is noticed by anyone. With these techniques, an impressive, confident look is always within your reach.

Last, I'd like to thank you for purchasing this book! If you enjoyed it or found it helpful, I'd greatly appreciate it if you'd take a moment to leave a review on Amazon. Thank you!

36564003R00031

Printed in Great Britain
by Amazon